Why Weight?

A Short Guide to Losing Weight Immediately

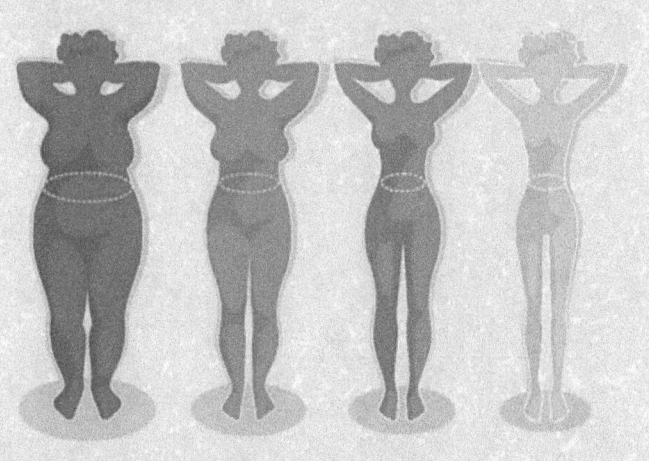

J.R. EADY

Legal Notice

Table of Contents

INTRODUCTION

I would like to thank you and congratulate you for purchasing this book. Being in the physical fitness field all of my adult life as a personal trainer, I have had the opportunity to train people from all walks of life seeking to lose weight including post-partum mothers. In this book, I will provide you with a simple method that has no gimmicks and works every time. I have personally used this method several times. The weight loss industry rakes in over a whopping $20 billion dollars annually! Diets are a fad and designed to fail. Why spend money aimlessly when you have had the ability all along?

This book will show you how. Weight loss should be an easy, straightforward process. Just as easy as we consume calories, we should also be able to expend them. You shouldn't be pressed, nervous, or afraid about losing pounds. Reaching your goal weight shouldn't be looked at as a task that is unachievable or costs thousands of dollars. There is no "magic pill" or secret exercise that will instantly allow you to lose weight; however, it is quite easy.

It all boils down to science. You will learn a method which has always been within your grasp. This method requires virtually no exercise but doing so will only increase your results exponentially. I would like you to affirm your weight loss goal before continuing and believe that it will come to pass by the time that you have completed this book. The body that you desire is waiting on you! Are you ready?

1:
WHAT IS WEIGHT?

Understanding Weight

To understand weight, we must fundamentally understand what the unit of measure we call a pound (lb) consists of. When we think about weight we generally think about calories. Well what exactly are calories besides numbers that we generally assign to food? Calories are units of heat energy that are found in foods and drinks that we consume. These are known as "large calories" or "kcals" which equals to the amount required to raise the temperature of 1 kilogram of water by 1 degree Celsius. Weight gain and weight loss boils down to the simple formula of calorie intake versus calorie output. Our daily lifestyle essentially reflects this based upon our activity levels. There are three levels of activity; sedentary, moderately active, and active. The higher the level of activity equates to the more calories that should be consumed based upon age and gender.

- Sedentary is a lifestyle with little to no physical activity.
- Being Moderately active is a lifestyle associated with walking 1.5 to 3 miles per day during daily activities.
- Active is a lifestyle associated with walking more than 3 miles per day during daily activities.

Most nutrition fact labels you find on food items are based upon a 2,000 calorie diet. This is an amount agreed upon by the FDA (1) in the United States of America. As I stated before, our age and gender determine how much calories we require to function on a daily basis. The only variable to this is our activity level. We should look at our bodies as machines that require fuel. The less work or activity the machine does, the less fuel is consumed hence less fuel is required. We are no different. If we live a sedentary lifestyle, we should not be consuming the same calories of one who is living an active lifestyle. Males require more calories than females due to the biological make up. This difference is normally between 200 and 400 calories on average depending on the age. Our activity level is normally on the increase from the time we are born until we reach our 30's and 40's.

In 2002, the Institute of Medicine (2) developed a system called the Estimated Energy Requirement (ERR) which predicts the average amount of calories a person would require to have a healthy weight. The EER is great for determining what you require but it is designed for what is considered "normal weight" individuals and is also based on activity level. My method is not exclusive to normal weight or activity level. But we will get into that later in this book.

One Pound

By now you are probably wondering, "Why do I need to know all of this?" That is quite understandable. I myself had to research to find what exactly is the root of this and why? I narrowed it down to the number that we all dread when hopping on the scale. Pounds. Many diet blogs, books, and experts will say that one pound is 3,500 calories. In fact this number can vary based upon the percentage of lipid in the fat tissue of your body. This number can actually be somewhere between 2,800 and 3,700 calories to equal a pound. With that in mind, I tend to shoot for the higher number to have the satisfaction that I am covered.

Our calories can be ultimately derived from three sources: Proteins, carbohydrates, and fats. These are known as macronutrients or macros as they are commonly known in dieting. The composition of your calories/pounds also affects weight loss. A balance of your daily macros is important for leading a healthy lifestyle. Your protein develops muscle, reduces hunger, and requires more calories to digest than the other two. Proteins require approximately 20-30% of it's total just to digest. This means that if you eat 100 calories of protein, you are really only getting 70-80 calories after digestion. This is amazing because it is a plus for consuming more proteins than any of the other two macros.

Carbohydrates are necessary for energy and sugar levels. Fats are necessary for hormone regulation, vitamin absorption and brain function. Proteins and carbohydrates each equal 4 calories for every 1 gram. One gram of fat equals 9 calories. This is useful for formulating eating plans and goal setting when aspiring to achieve a specific body type. Because of the important functions that each of these macros serve, there should be a balance and moderate percentage of each in your diet.

Why is this important? This is important to set a quantifiable number that we can target when implementing a method to lose weight. Our goal is lose excess and unwanted fat while maintaining our muscle. A common myth that you may also have heard is that muscle weighs more that fat. This is about as true as the thought that calories from fruit are different from calories from a cheeseburger. A calorie is a calorie. A pound of fat weighs the same as a pound of muscle, lead, sand, or jello. A pound is a pound. 16 ounces. 454 grams. The difference between muscle and fat is the density and volume. Muscle is more dense and has less volume than fat. Muscle also burns more calories when your body is at rest. That is why exercise is important but it is not necessary to lose weight. It just expedites the process and acts as a catalyst.

2:
YOUR BODY IN TRANSITION

Body Mass Index[BMI]

Your Body Mass Index or BMI (3) is a formula that is used to determine a healthy weight. This does not necessarily mean that you are in bad health or good health based upon this formula. However, this formula reflects if you are overweight or obese which can lead to health problems such as breathing problems, high blood pressure, heart disease, type 2 diabetes, gallstones, and certain cancers. Due to our genetics and family history, some of these health problems are unavoidable but we can mitigate some of these by maintaining a healthy weight. Don't ever believe that you were predisposed to be a certain weight due to genetics or family history. You are in control! Below you will find an example of a BMI chart.

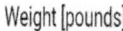

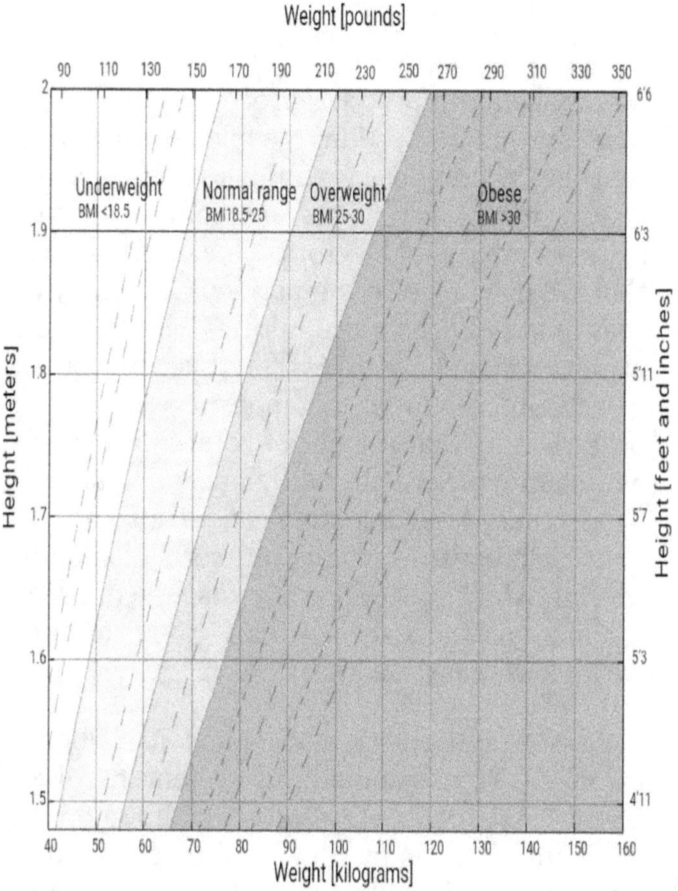
Weight [pounds]
90 110 130 150 170 190 210 230 250 270 290 310 330 350
Underweight
BMI <18.5
Normal range
BMI18.5-25
Overweight
BMI 25-30
Obese
BMI >30
Height [meters]
2 1.9 1.8 1.7 1.6 1.5
Height [feet and inches]
6'6 6'3 5'11 5'7 5'3 4'11
40 50 60 70 80 90 100 110 120 130 140 150 160
Weight [kilograms]

Metabolism and Fasting

Metabolism is our body's process of converting food into energy. Many people tend to think that they cannot lose weight because they have a slow metabolism. This isn't completely true as there are several factors. One of the factors that we discussed in the previous chapter was that muscle burns more calories when you are at rest. If you have excess fat, this contributes directly to a slower metabolism. There are other factors that are out of your control such as an underactive thyroid gland or Cushing's syndrome. Your age and gender also affects your metabolism but this ultimately is due to muscle which we previously discussed. Men tend to have more muscle than women and yet we all lose muscle as we age.

Digestion and energy conversion itself burns calories. This is something we tend to forget about. We consume foods and initiate this mechanical action by chewing food or drinking and then swallowing. Once the food reaches the stomach the chemical processes begin. This action processes, absorbs, stores and burns calories which is known as thermogenesis. Other body processes that we overlook as part of our metabolism that burn calories passively and involuntarily are breathing, blood circulation, repairing cells, and thousands of others that we are oblivious to. Even while we are sleeping we are burning calories! The body is a 24/7 operating machine that requires fuel to function. That fuel is constantly burning whether we are conscious of it or not.

Fasting has been prescribed for thousands of years by doctors, spiritual leaders, and in religious scripture of different faiths around the world. There are numerous benefits of fasting and the most obvious one is weight loss. Fasting is a natural way of detoxifying the body and evening out hormone levels. This body "reset" also initiates cell repair and reduces stress and inflammation. Fasting intermittently initiates fat burning quickly. When done properly, it will cause you to eat less and have fewer meals. This is in part due to the stomach being adjusted to digesting less food over time. Intermittent fasting can be done by abstaining from food and drink for certain amount of time. For those just starting it can be rough the first couple of times. I recommend fasting two days out of the week at a period of at least two thirds of the day. This isn't quite as difficult as you would think. On average most of us sleep for eight hours a day. That's one third of a day right there! Add another third to this and this can lead to surprising results.

It is easier to enter into fat burning mode as you have already tapped into your carbohydrate storage (glycogen) and used them up for those 8 hours. Your body prefers to use carbs as a fuel source over fat. Technically, you have two fuel tanks so to speak; Carbohydrates can be considered your primary fuel tank and fat is your secondary fuel tank. Carbohydrates burn more quickly and are readily available while fats burn more efficiently because they contain more calories than carbohydrates. I like to use the similes that carbohydrates are like gasoline while fat is like diesel. To get to the diesel you must burn through all of your gasoline. The primary fuel source must be depleted before tapping into the secondary. That is the goal! If your glycogen storage is not used as energy, it is then converted into fat. Our bodies are designed to store fat in preparation for times that food may not be readily available. Based on the percentage of body fat we have, there are thousands of calories stored to be used for energy as we have discussed earlier. Our bodies will essentially feed off of these fat calories by burning them. This process is called ketosis.

During the time following breaking the fast, one should abstain from binging just to make up for missed meals. It is not required, and I will discuss this later in the book. Many people think of fasting as not eating or drinking anything for an entire day. This is not true. Remember, fasting can be accomplished by just abstaining from food and beverage for a substantial part of the day. Fasting can also be accomplished by just drinking liquids for a certain time period. There are numerous ways of doing it. What you should not do is starve yourself without sustenance daily. You will still have to maintain a health nutrition level to function properly.

Exercise and Waste Elimination

First off, I wanted to say that I am a firm believer in exercise and physical fitness. However, for the purpose of this book, I want to let you know that it is not required to lose weight. It is definitely a positive and can accelerate your weight loss process tremendously when combined with the method in this book. We are at different points in our lives in terms of levels of physical fitness and some may not be as capable as others and may even be unable to exercise. For those who are capable, simply taking a short walk or engaging in a light activity for 10 minutes a few times throughout the day can burn calories quickly. Things as simple as sweeping, mopping, rearranging furniture, or cleaning all the windows in your home can become a routine workout. The possibilities are endless. The goal is to remain active throughout your day. Don't be afraid to sweat. There are numerous apps that can be downloaded to track your progress throughout the day. There are apps that track your steps, distance walked, and estimated calories burned while sleeping and relaxing. Look for some of these apps and you will be surprised at the results and information you find about your daily activities.

We have discussed calories, weight, metabolism and exercise, but one thing I have noticed that is rarely discussed in weight loss blogs, magazines, and by personnel is waste elimination. This is the byproduct of consuming food and drink. The process of waste elimination rids our bodies of both liquids and solids containing toxins, undigested food, and vitamins and minerals that we do not require. This is crucial because this ultimately affects our weight loss on a more passive scale that we normally would not think of. We rid our bodies of waste by sweating, breathing, urinating, and defecating. We often believe that we just consume the food, thermogenesis is initiated and everything is forgotten. Not so fast. Much more continues to happen during the digestion process. Breathing, sweating, and urinating all eliminate waste without absorbing nutrients and calories. Defecation, or bowel movement, is a more complex process

After the food arrives in our stomachs and is further broken down into liquid or paste by stomach acid and other enzymes, it moves on into the small intestine. Digestion continues here where enzymes are released by the pancreas and bile is released by the liver to break down fat and eliminate waste. Calories and nutrients are still being absorbed during this stage. After this point, whatever food is left is then moved to your large intestine also known as your colon. While in the colon, the food is formed into a stool. The stool is composed of food debris and bacteria. Within the colon is its own ecosystem of bacteria - both beneficial and harmful. The longer the stool remains in the colon the more vitamins, nutrients, and calories are absorbed. The intestines play a huge part in our immune system. If anything goes wrong in our intestines, it has the potential to affect all of our major organs adversely.

Why do I mention all of this? The answer is simple: Effective stool evacuation. Having an effective stool evacuation is key to maintaining a great metabolism. Our digestive system should be seamless in its operation - similar to a conveyor belt. If one of the sections gets blocked, it affects the

entire belt. From the time that we are born, our digestive system functions naturally without any hesitation. We eat and then have a bowel movement when the urge comes. As we grow older, we have conditioned ourselves to delay our bowel movement until we find the right accommodation to accomplish the task. This is not natural. This can have an adverse effect such as constipation which can lead to many other colorectal disorders. The overwhelming medical advice will suggest that you have a bowel movement once every three days and this is considered normal. The fourth day would make you amongst those who are considered constipated. Ideally, for a healthy digestive system and metabolism, you should have a bowel movement after every large meal if not daily. The key to this is to have an adequate amount of dietary fat to stimulate intestinal motility. The other two macronutrients, protein and carbohydrates, have no effect on it.

However, fiber, which is a carbohydrate, acts as a sponge pushing thru your intestines absorbing water, bacteria, and waste. It also adds bulk to your stool. This brings me to my last point of eliminating waste. One gram of carbohydrates requires approximately 3-4 grams of water to be stored in our bodies. This becomes an issue when we consume a high carb meal. For example, we consume a meal that contains 112 carbs, that will require 12-16 ounces of water to store in your body. That is approximately an additional pound in water retained from that meal! This is where the term "water weight" comes from. This is also why many of you may have heard that carbs are bad. Everything is fine in moderation and carbs can be used to accomplish certain fitness goals. But that is a whole other topic. Waste elimination via bowel movement is one of the most efficient ways of accomplishing weight loss as it completes the digestion. Sweating and breathing remove the excess water being stored between your cells and tissue. Urinating should come natural as long as you continue to ingest fluids, barring you having a health condition. Be conscious of all of this. You are in control.

Water Weight

Another factor which you have probably heard about is the water weight that we carry with us daily. The amount of this weight can vary drastically based upon our diet. The main two factors in our diet that contribute to water weight is our carbohydrate and sodium intake. Also a lack of water or dehydration can cause water retention as well. First we will discuss carbohydrates and then sodium and how their relationship affects us with water retention.

Our body chemistry is designed in such a way that when we consume one gram of carbs it requires 3-4 grams of water just to store it. This can add up quickly when you are consuming a high carb meal. For example, let's say you ate a pasta and breadsticks meal which totaled about 100 grams in carbs. In the worst case that would equal to about 400 grams of water. There are 28 grams in an ounce so let's do a little math.

400 grams / 28 grams = 14 ounces of water

That is almost a pound of water weight from one meal! The same holds true for sodium, or salt as we commonly refer to it. Sodium requires water and retains it to balance the ration in our blood so our bodies function properly. The FDA recommends 2,300 milligrams a day of sodium. This is important to watch out for because sodium is stored in so many of the foods we eat. Sometimes we find food items that are low in calories, sugar, and fat but may be loaded in sodium to add flavor to the product. It is important to ration your sodium intake based upon your activity level. Things such as perspiration and urination regularly remove sodium from our body. The best way to resolve the issue of water weight due to sodium is to maintain low sodium levels, proper hydration and flushing our systems. We should be drinking about half an ounce of water for every pound that we weigh. So if you weigh 200 lbs you should be drinking around 100 ounces of water a day.

3:
THE METHOD

The Secret

By now, you are probably wondering when you are going to get to the part that tells you how to lose weight. Well that time has come. It is actually very simple. This is science, and as I have said before, your body is a machine. A perfect, complex product of divine engineering that cannot be duplicated. What you put in is what you get out. Since the dawn of mankind, we have been active hunters and gatherers. Food has not been always readily available the way it is now for many of us. Since the advent of fossil fuel, the engine, and then the industrial revolution, the world's population has skyrocketed due to the ability to create and harvest an abundance of food. This has also allowed us to distribute food throughout the world. This has lead to an abundance of processed sugar and obesity throughout the world. We eat more than we should simply because it is easily accessible. We are entitled to live abundantly but health wise we should be moderate when it comes to food consumption. There is a secret that I am ready to give you and you can still eat whatever you want......in moderation!

Through testing this "secret" on myself several times successfully as well as others, I have come up with a formula that works. The secret is based on a number that you want. What is the exact weight that you would like to be? Write it down. Now let's begin!

Let's say your number was 190 lbs. We can now take 190 and multiply it times 10. Or we can just make it easier and just add a 0 on the end of your number. So for example, your number will now become 1900. This number is now your official daily calorie intake also known as your secret. So how does this work? Well 1,900 calories is your Recommended Daily Intake or RDI. Your RDI enables you to reach your goal weight effectively and in an easy manner. This essentially creates a daily calorie deficit that doesn't require exercise. The larger the gap is between your weight and your goal weight, the faster you will lose weight. Because your body may have become so used to a certain amount of calories, this change will bring about quick weight loss. I liken this to, without comparing you to it, the diet plan or RDI that is given to morbidly obese patients before they are granted a gastric bypass surgery or similar stomach capacity reduction surgery. Many of these patients are given an RDI which is a difference of 1,000 plus less than what they are used to consuming. For example, if the patient weighs around 620 lbs, the doctor may prescribe them a RDI of 4,500 calories. Once they begin this diet, the pounds drop off effortlessly. Remember how many calories I said equals a pound? Keep that in mind. This caloric deficit may seem like quite the challenge but once you start you will find yourself not consuming as much as you usually would. The feeling of hunger or satiation will gradual decrease. This has been described by many as "stomach shrinking" feeling. Your eyes play a major part in how much you consume. I will describe this later in the chapter along with other tips that will get you successfully on your way to shedding pounds. Please don't forget to consult a physician to ensure that you are clear to proceed with this RDI or if you have a health issue(s) that may require a certain diet.

Nutrition Fact Labels

Nutrition Fact Labels are some of the most overlooked keys of information on food items. How many of us actually read them? Do we know what we are actually putting in our bodies? I have ran into so many people who don't actually take the time to or really don't care about it. A fraction of those who do read the labels don't actually read them properly. These labels are the blueprint of what the rest of your day will consist of and they can literally destroy your diet! A detail as simple as the Serving Size holds the key to macros and overall calories that could be overlooked. For the purpose of weight loss, we will focus on the macros and sodium. The most important macro that directly contributes to weight gain is carbohydrates. Carbohydrates break down into glucose which increases your blood sugar when you consume them. A high blood sugar level initiates the secretion of the hormone insulin from your pancreas. This spike of insulin lowers your blood sugar by forcing the sugar into your fat cells causing weight gain. If you are going to consume carbohydrates, do it in moderation. Consume complex carbs over processed carbs if possible. Complex carbs are whole grains, green vegetables, and fruits.

Below you will find 2 Nutrition Fact Labels. The first label is a can of tuna. I listed tuna because it is easily one of highest sources of protein that you can get with minimal calories. Canned tuna comes in different varieties and is very inexpensive. On the label you will see that there is a total of 3 Servings at 80 calories per Serving. That equals a total of 240 calories for the whole can. Since there are 3 servings you will multiply every macro by 3 to get the total amount that you are actually getting in this can.

Nutrition Facts

Serving Size 1 can drained (62g)
Servings Per Container 3 Cans
Calories 80
   Calories from Fat 25

Amount / Serving	% Daily Value*	Amount / Serving	% Daily Value*
Total Fat 2.5g	4%	Sodium 200mg	8%
Saturated Fat 0g	0%	Potassium 100mg	3%
Trans Fat 0g		Total Carbohydrate 0g	0%
Polyunsaturated Fat 1.5g		Dietary Fiber 0g	0%
Monounsaturated Fat 0.5g		Sugars 0g	
Cholesterol 30mg	10%	Protein 12g	22%

Vitamin A 0%	• Vitamin C 0%	Calcium 2%	• Iron 2%
Vitamin D 8%	• Niacin 20%	Vitamin B6 6%	• Vitamin B12 25%
Selenium 45%			

The next label below is that of your typical soft drink. I listed a soft drink because this is one of the items that many people consume on a daily basis and think nothing of it. Many of us actually consume several in a day. On this label you can see that it is a total of 2.5 Servings per bottle at 110 calories per Serving. That equals to 275 calories per bottle. A 20 ounce bottle. Now let's take a look at the carbohydrates. That equals a total of 93 grams of carbohydrates. So with the understanding that we are ingesting 93 grams of carbohydrates, we can find out how much water weight we will be taking on along with that based off of what we have learned earlier. There are 4 grams of water for every 1 gram of carbohydrates so that leaves us with a total of 372 grams of water. We divide 372 grams of water by 28 to get our ounces which is rounded down to 13 ounces. That is just 3 ounces shy of a pound! So by drinking this beverage it will require 13 ounces of water just to store it! Incredible!

Nutrition Facts

Serving Size 8 fl oz (240 mL)
Servings Per Container 2.5

Amount Per Serving

Calories 110

% Daily Value*

Total Fat 0g	**0%**
Sodium 50mg	**2%**
Total Carbohydrate 31g	**10%**
Sugars 31g	
Protein 0g	

Foods, Diet, and Tips

In this section I will be discussing a few things that will place you on your way to weight loss success. These tips that I will be giving you have come from research and trial and error. There is no "broscience" in this- just fundamentals that will aid in reaching your goal. As I said before, if you choose to begin this process you must affirm this and will it into existence. Discipline is the first key. Everything else will fall in place. So to start off:

- ❖ Again, have DISCIPLINE! Think of the end goal.
- ❖ Set your calorie count at whatever your goal weight is by adding a 0 at the end of it. Example goal weight is 150 lbs so that would make your calorie count 1500 calories.
- ❖ Limit your beverages to water only. Consume half an ounce of water per pound of your body weight.
- ❖ Drink ice cold water. Distilled water if possible. Your body will burn more

calories to warm it up to your internal temperature once you drink it.

- ❖ A natural fat flush, detox, and diuretic that you can make is by adding slices of lemon and oranges to your water. This will flush out the fat and promote frequent urination to rid your body of excess sodium and waste. Be sure to add an electrolyte like potassium while using this.

- ❖ Use diuretics to promote water weight loss. There are natural diuretics and vegan pills that are available for purchase online or at your local pharmacy.

- ❖ When you prepare to eat be mindful of what you put on your plate. Your eyes will encourage you to continue eating past the point that you are actually full. Do not eat until you are FULL.

- ❖ Sit down and eat your meals. Chew slowly. If you are still hungry after you have finished your meal, wait 5-10 minutes and the hunger will subside.

- ❖ When you consume a meal, the contents of your stomach should be one third water, one third food, and one third air.

- ❖ Liquid calories such as soda, juices, and milk can easily make up one third to half of your daily calorie intake.

- For quicker weight loss focus on a high protein, mid to high fat, and low carbohydrate diet.
- Carbohydrates in your diet should be complex such as whole grains, oats, fruits and green vegetables.
- Avoid excess sugars and artificial sweeteners.
- Weight gain can essentially be linked to hormones. Insulin is a hormone secreted by the pancreas in reaction to an increase in blood sugar levels due to the consumption of carbs. The insulin spikes pushing the glucose from the carbs into your fat cells to lower your blood sugar level. This essentially causes weight gain in a nutshell.
- Try to cook your meals if possible and season them with spices to boost your metabolism.
- Take a fiber supplement such as psyllium husks and senegal acacia to keep the digestive system moving. Fiber grams do not count towards your total carbohydrates count because it is indigestible and you cannot get energy from them.
- Try to bulk up your meals by adding quantities of green veggies such as lettuce, spinach, kale and cabbage. They

have virtually no calories and fill you up quick while offering other health benefits.

❖ Caffeine is an appetite suppressant. Use that to your benefit.

❖ Fast for two thirds of your day twice a week. If two thirds is too difficult, try half a day. Remember that the time that you are asleep counts!

❖ Exercise immediately after waking up or after a short fast to go directly into fat burning mode. Even if it is a walk or light calisthenics.

❖ Stay active throughout your day. The more focused you are and the less amount of idle time you have, the less likely you are to snack or binge on food.

❖ Fat does not burn in one targeted spot. It burns throughout the body all at once. Tailor your exercises to working different parts of the bod y. **The largest muscle group in the body is in your legs. Keep that in mind. **hint****

❖ When exercising exert yourself until your body feels slightly warm and you have labored breathing.

❖ If possible use the sauna a couple of times a week for a natural detox and for water weight loss. If you don't have a sauna, you can create a makeshift one by filling a tub with hot water as hot as you can stand and sit in it for 15-20 minutes. You can also close the door to your bathroom and place a towel at the bottom of the door. Turn on your shower to a temperature that is hot enough for you to stand in and do the same for 15-20 minutes.

❖   Have fun!

PARTING WORDS

At this point of closing I enjoin that you all proceed in your new endeavor with a fun an optimistic approach. You now have the tools to reach your desired goal. This process should be done in a relaxed, stress free manner making every time that you step on the scale like Christmas morning receiving gifts. Your gift is your progress as you watch the numbers dwindle on your scale. You are on a path to a healthier lifestyle that can completely change your life. Your health and well being is one of those things that you cannot purchase and yet it takes no special skill to get in shape. You walk around daily as the pilot of a complex machine that is composed of a combination of chemical reactions and a vast circuit board of neuroelectric synapses. You are a natural thermogenerator capable of producing 330 Body Temperature Units (BTUs) per hour on average. That is enough to power a 100-watt light bulb for an hour! This is the passive ability that you possess. Do you remember what the source of this passive ability is?

Calories: Your body's energy source measured in heat.

You are in control and you possess the keys to unlocking the door that may be blocking you. Do not become discouraged and if you begin to feel that way just remember why you started. You set the pace on how quickly you want the results. There is no competition except yourself from yesterday. Everyday is a new opportunity to take the step that you may have been going over in your mind. Why wait? Do it now. Best of wishes on your journey and may peace and happiness be upon you!

FOR MORE ON J.R. EADY

Facebook: Hyperbolic Fitness & Nutrition | @jayrwisdom

Instagram: poetically_scripted

YouTube: Hyperbolic Fitness

For all general questions.

For customized meal plans contact hyperbolicfitness1@gmail.com.

BIBLIOGRAPHY

1. "How to Understand and Use the Nutrition Facts." *U.S. Food and Drug Administration*, FDA, 14 July 2015. www.fda.gov . 23 June 2016

2. "Institute of Medicine - Estimated Energy Requirement (EER)." *GlobalRph*, GlobalRph, 10 March 2016. Www.globalrph.com. 23 June 2016

3. "Body Mass Index." *Body Mass Index*, Wikipedia, 1 July 2016. En.wikipedia.org. 23 June 2016